THE NEW CARNIVORE

Cookbook

High-protein carnivore recipes, Paleo Carnivore Cooking guide, Zero-carb carnivore meals

Table of contents

INTRODUCTION

Amid trendy diets promising health and weight loss, interest in radical carnivore and all-meat eating plans has been gaining steam. Eliminating plant foods and deriving nourishment solely from animal sources appeals to those seeking reduced inflammation, improved digestion, lower food sensitivities, and control of chronic conditions from autoimmunity to mood disorders. However, such an extreme dietary approach naturally raises questions and skepticism. In this cookbook, we aim to explore the theoretical benefits of carnivore eating along with practical guidance for following the diet safely long-term, including approachable recipes utilizing meat, eggs, and low-carb dairy to make this restrictive regimen more enjoyable and sustainable.

Chapter 1:

The idea of an all-meat diet, or carnivore diet, often raises eyebrows or skepticism at first mention. Eating only animal foods seems extreme in today's world of veganism and plant-based lifestyles. However, the carnivore diet has recently been growing in popularity among health-conscious consumers looking to lose weight, reduce inflammation, and improve chronic disease conditions.

What is a Carnivore Diet?

A carnivore diet, as its name implies, consists of eating only animal foods and eliminating all plants from the diet. The staples tend to be red meat, poultry, fish, eggs, and dairy like butter or heavy cream. Some variations may include or omit dairy. The carnivore diet is made up entirely of protein, fat, and nutrients found naturally in animal foods. All fruits, vegetables, grains, legumes, nuts, seeds, plant-based oils, and sugars are excluded.

Water, tea, and coffee are acceptable beverages on a carnivore diet. Some people may also include small amounts of seasonings, spices, vinegars, and fermented foods as long as they do not contain added sugars or carbohydrates. The carnivore diet is naturally low in carbohydrates, high in protein, and moderate to high in fat. This macros ratio puts the body into a state of ketosis, similar to the ketogenic diet.

Brief History of the Carnivore Diet

Eating an all-meat diet goes back to prehistoric times when hunter-gatherer groups subsisted on animals they hunted and fish they caught. However, the modern carnivore diet trend seems to have emerged in the last decade through influences like the low-carb, paleo, and keto movements.

In 2010, Swedish doctor Annika Dahlqvist began recommending a low-carb, high-fat diet to her patients with obesity, diabetes, and digestive issues. She found that many improved simply by eliminating plants and sugar. Around this same time, Canadian osteopath Shawn Baker adopted a carnivore eating style and reported better health and athletic performance.

The diet gained wider recognition in 2018 when clinical psychologist Jordan Peterson and his daughter Mikhaila documented their experiences eating only beef, salt, and water for health purposes. Since then, the carnivore diet has been growing in popularity thanks to podcasts, social media groups, Reddit forums, and word-of-mouth.

Claimed Health Benefits of a Carnivore Diet

Advocates of the carnivore diet point to many potential health benefits, though more research is still needed:

Weight loss - The high protein and fat keeps appetite and cravings suppressed leading to easier calorie restriction for weight loss.

Reduced inflammation - Animal foods contain no lectins, phytates, or anti-nutrients that can cause intestinal inflammation like some plants.

Improved digestion - The carnivore diet is typically easy to digest and can relieve gastrointestinal issues.

Increased energy - Lack of carbs eliminates blood sugar crashes. The diet provides steady energy from protein and fat.

Mental clarity - Ketosis and stable blood sugar provide enhanced focus and cognitive function.

Blood sugar control - The absence of carbs prevents spikes in blood glucose levels. It may help manage diabetes.

Heart health - Increased intake of omega-3s found in fatty fish while limiting carbs and omega-6s.

Skin improvements - Some see reductions in eczema, acne, or skin conditions without plant-based trigger foods.

Autoimmune regulation - Lack of gut irritation can calm autoimmune responses for some people.

Allergy relief - Eliminating common allergens like grains, legumes, nuts, seeds and nightshade vegetables.

Of course, individual results will vary based on your personal health history. Some may experience improvements in certain areas, while others may not see any noticeable changes. Monitoring key biomarkers before and during the diet can help you gauge any effects.

Potential Concerns and Considerations

Such an extreme way of eating naturally raises some questions and doubts. Here are some common concerns:

Lack of fiber - Without plant foods, digestive regularity may become an issue. Some carnivores report improvement, while others admit occasional constipation. Staying hydrated and eating plenty of fat helps. Digestive enzymes or probiotic supplements can also aid gut function.

Nutrient deficiencies - Critics claim essential vitamins and minerals found mostly in plants will be missing. However, animal foods also provide complete proteins, B12, iron, zinc, selenium. Moderate organ meats consumption also provides nutrients like Vitamin A. Still, consulting a doctor is wise, especially for those with conditions requiring special nutrient needs.

Increased cancer risk - Some data shows increased colon cancer risk with excessive red meat intake. However, the association is unclear. Lean meats, lifestyle factors, and plant toxins may also play a role. More research on long-term carnivore diets is needed.

Kidney problems - Kidneys filter nitrogenous waste from animal protein. Those with chronic kidney disease may need to limit protein. Healthy kidneys have been shown to easily adapt to higher protein intakes. But it's wise to monitor kidney function when significantly increasing protein.

Cardiovascular concerns - Saturated fats raise blood cholesterol for some people, increasing heart disease risk. But studies show fat quality matters more than quantity. Omega-3 fats, monounsaturated fats, and low-oxidized cholesterol in fresh meat may reduce inflammation and plaque buildup.

Microbiome diversity - Plant fibers feed gut bacteria that produce beneficial compounds and vitamins. Drastically reducing carb intake can decrease microbial diversity over time. Periodic higher-fiber meals, prebiotics, or probiotics may help counteract this.

Listening to your body and discussing any health changes with your doctor is important when making major diet shifts. Testing blood work at intervals can also detect potential nutritional shortcomings.

Starting a Carnivore Diet

Now that we've covered the basics, let's discuss how to start a carnivore diet:

Prep your kitchen - Remove non-carnivore pantry items. Stock up on red meat, poultry, fish, eggs, ghee, tallow, heavy cream and any approved spices. Shop from quality sources if possible.

Cut carbs gradually - Eliminating all carbs abruptly may cause cravings or energy dips initially. Try gradually tapering down carbs over 2-4 weeks for an easier adaptation.

Stay hydrated - Drink plenty of non-sweetened beverages. Dehydration causes headaches, fogginess, and constipation. Aim for at least 2 liters of water daily. Adding electrolytes can help.

Eat when hungry - Listen to your body's signals. Appetite typically decreases the longer you are fat-adapted. Eat more or less based on hunger, not fixed meal times.

Increase fat intake - Getting adequate fat helps keep energy levels stable, control hunger, and aids vitamin absorption. Include fatty cuts of meat, high-fat dairy, tallow, butter, and bone marrow.

Get enough calories - If you lose weight rapidly, increase your calorie intake. Very low-calorie diets can cause side effects. Stabilizing your weight prevents heavy ketosis.

Supplement if needed - Some may benefit from digestive enzymes, probiotics, electrolyte supplements to start. Discuss any other supplements with your doctor.

Reintroduce limited carbs/plants if needed - If you experience constipation, cravings, hormonal issues or fatigue, try adding small amounts of carbs back in before quitting. Tubers, fruit, rice or potatoes are best-tolerated options.

The adaptation period lasts 2-6 weeks as your body gets used to burning fat rather than glucose for fuel. Symptoms like low energy, sugar cravings, headaches, dizziness or gastrointestinal issues tend to resolve within a few weeks for most people.

Ways to Thrive on a Carnivore Diet

Here are some tips for feeling your best on a long-term carnivore diet:

Seek variety within the carnivore parameters. Alternate different protein sources like beef, lamb, bison, seafood, pork and poultry. Try organ meats like liver or brain occasionally for micronutrients and variety.

Pay attention to fat quality. Focus on high omega-3 choices like grass-fed beef, fatty fish and pasture-raised eggs whenever possible. Avoid highly processed meats.

Drink bone broth for collagen and hydration. Bone broth provides gelatin, electrolytes, and minerals. Sipping it throughout the day prevents dehydration.

Make meals appetizing. Turn to spices, pan drippings, or xanthan gum to create sauces and seasonings. Sear or dry rub meats for that satisfying umami, Maillard reaction flavor.

Find community support. Join social media groups, forums and podcasts to connect with others following a carnivore lifestyle. They can provide meal inspiration, accountability and reassurance.

Monitor labs and symptoms. Schedule regular blood work to watch biomarkers. Also track subjective symptoms like energy, sleep, cognition, mood

Chapter 2:

Sourcing Quality Meats

The foundation of any carnivore diet is access to high-quality protein sources. When meat makes up the entirety of your diet, sourcing becomes especially important. Not all meat is created equal, with factors like farming practices, processing methods, and cut selection all affecting nutritional content and health value. This chapter covers how to identify and obtain top-tier animal foods to thrive on an all-meat lifestyle.

Understanding Meat Quality

Meat quality depends largely on how the source animal was raised and fed. Conventionally raised, factory-farmed meat offers lower quality while still costing less per pound. However, higher quality options maximize nutrients while minimizing inflammatory compounds.

Feed: Grass-fed cows or pasture-raised chickens eat a natural, species-appropriate diet. This results in higher antioxidant levels and better fatty acid profiles. Grain-fed animals contain more pro-inflammatory omega-6s.

Living conditions: Access to fresh air, space to roam, and low-stress handling creates healthier animals. Crowded, confined factory farm conditions lead to more disease and infections.

Drug use: Conventional farms rely heavily on antibiotics and hormones to accelerate growth. Hormones are banned in chicken, but prevalent in cattle. Residues can negatively impact human hormones and gut health.

Processing: Opt for minimally processed cuts without preservatives or additives like nitrites. Dry aged meat also enhances flavor and tenderness naturally via enzymes.

Grass-fed versus Grain-fed Meat

Grass-fed meat comes from cows, bison, lamb, and other ruminants fed a natural diet of grass rather than cereal grains. Grass-fed meat offers higher nutritional value than conventional, grain-fed meat in the following ways:

More omega-3 fatty acids - Grass-fed meat contains 2-4X higher levels of anti-inflammatory omega-3s compared to grain-fed. This creates a healthier ratio of omega-6 to omega-3 fatty acids.

Higher antioxidant levels - Grass-fed meat provides more antioxidant compounds like vitamin E, beta-carotene, superoxide dismutase and glutathione. These help combat oxidative stress.

More micronutrients - Meat from grass-fed animals contains higher amounts of nutrients like iron, zinc, phosphorus, B vitamins, selenium and calcium.

Improved flavor - Grass-fed meat tends to have a richer, beefier, more complex taste from the diverse grass diet. Marbling fat also takes on a healthier yellow hue.

Less external toxins - Pasture-raised animals take in fewer pesticides, heavy metals, and pollutants compared to factory farm feedlot animals. Toxins accumulate in fat cells.

Fewer antibiotics/hormones - Grass-fed farms use fewer drugs and antibiotics to prevent disease compared to crowded feedlots. No added hormones avoids endocrine disruption.

More CLA and bioactive compounds - Grass-fed meat contains more conjugated linoleic acid and other bioactive agents that provide anticancer and anti-inflammatory benefits in studies.

Finding and Budgeting for Grass-Fed Meat

The main downside of grass-fed meat tends to be the higher cost compared to conventional options. However, the price difference is narrowing as it gains mainstream popularity. Here are some tips for finding affordable grass-fed meat:

Check local farms - Buying direct from local ranches that grass-feed can offer bulk deals on mixed quarter or half cow purchases. You can also ensure authenticity.

Join a CSA (community supported agriculture) program - Pay upfront to receive regular deliveries of meat, eggs, dairy and produce from small regional farms.

Look for mark-downs - Meat nearing its sell-by date is often marked down up to 50%. Stock up and freeze extra bargains.

Seek out wholesale clubs - Wholesale warehouse clubs like Costco now sell certified grass-fed beef in bulk for 20-30% cheaper.

Buy in bulk online - Reputable online vendors like Butcher Box deliver frozen grass-fed meat in bulk for about $5-8/lb for variety pack bundles.

Purchase fattier cuts - Ribeyes, brisket, chuck shoulder steaks offer more nutrition ounce for your dollar compared to lean sirloins or **tenderloins.**

Eat budget-friendly meats too - Alternate grass-fed varieties with pasture-raised chicken, eggs, pork and wild-caught canned fish.

Make it stretch as leftovers - Use marinades, slow cookers, and sauces to repurpose leftovers into new entrees. Bone broth simmers turn scraps into stock.

If grass-fed varieties remain cost-prohibitive, grain-finished is still preferable to feedlot meat. Seek the best quality your circumstances allow.

Decoding Meat & Poultry Labels

With so many buzzwords like natural, organic, free-range, and more on meat labels, it can get confusing decoding which terms truly signal better quality:

100% Grass-Fed: By law, cows eat only grass after being weaned from mother's milk. No grains ever. This is the gold standard for beef.

Grass-fed, Grain-finished: Cows eat grass the majority of life but get supplementary grains for the last few months. Still an improvement over straight grain-fed.

Pasture-raised: Indicates animals had access to outdoor spaces to roam somewhat freely. No real legal definition so verify source.

Organic: Mandates no antibiotics, hormones or GMOs used. Feed must be organic but not necessarily grass only.

Natural: Very loosely defined by USDA. Still allows some drug and hormone use. Minimal processing but not verified.

Free-range: Applies to poultry meaning birds had some access to the outdoors. Does not necessarily indicate quality of feed or living conditions.

Cage-free: For eggs, means hens are not confined to small individual cages but does not guarantee access outdoors.

Hormone-free: Can only be applied to poultry as hormones are not allowed at all for chickens, turkeys etc.

Reading up on common label claims and knowing trusted certifications like American Grassfed can help avoid misleading marketing. If unsure, call the producer to ask detailed questions.

Choosing Quality Cuts of Meat

Beyond the farming practices, meat quality also depends on which cuts and varieties you select. Follow these tips for picking optimal cuts:

Focus on whole primal and sub primal cuts rather than pre-made ground meat which oxidizes faster. Purchase whole steaks, roasts, chops etc.

Look for nicely marbled cuts which indicate healthy saturated and monounsaturated fat content throughout the muscle rather than just surface fat.

For beef, choose fattier cuts like ribeye, brisket, chuck shoulder, short ribs. Avoid leaner cuts like sirloin, round, tenderloin.

For pork, pick fattier cuts like belly, shoulder, ribs, butt/Boston butt. Avoid ultra lean tenderloin or "other white meat".

For poultry, choose skin-on thighs and legs over breast meat. The skin contains healthy fats and nutrients the muscles don't.

When possible, choose thicker, well-marbled heritage breed pork like Berkshire, Red Wattle or Mangalitsa for superior flavor and nutrition.

For lamb, stick to rendered cuts like shoulder, ribs, shank and leg instead of loin or chops which tend to be pricier.

With wild game like venison, elk, boar, and bison, marinating more strongly flavored cuts can help balance taste.

Additionally, the following varieties provide nutritional superstars:

Liver is one of the most nutrient-dense foods available, loaded with bioavailable vitamin A, B vitamins, iron, choline and more.

Bone marrow provides dense minerals like magnesium, phosphorus, selenium and easily absorbed collagen protein.

Heart and other organ meats offer huge amounts of minerals, cofactors like CoQ10, and superfood compounds for minimal calories.

Oily fish like sardines, anchovies, herring, trout and wild salmon provide anti-inflammatory omega-3 fatty acids.

Butchering for Affordability

Purchasing whole primal cuts like briskets, sirloin tips and pork bellies to butcher yourself saves considerably over pre-cut steaks and chops from the meat case. You also gain more control over portioning. A few helpful tools include:

Butcher's knife or cleaver: Look for full tang high-carbon steel blades. Can last generations if properly sharpened and honed.

Meat grinder: Lets you freshly grind roasts into ground meat as needed for peak flavor and nutrition. Great for making homemade sausage also.

Food processor: Useful for chopping and grinding smaller meat batches quicker. Especially helpful pulverizing liver for paté.

Meat slicer: Allows you to thinly slice roasts for deli-style lunches with zero effort. Ideal for carving roast beef or porchetta evenly.

Vacuum sealer: After portioning large cuts, vacuum seal extras for max freezer shelf life. Prevents freezer burn or oxidation

Chapter 3:

Beef Recipes

Beef forms the cornerstone of many carnivore diets thanks to its stellar nutrition profile and hearty, savory taste. From quick weeknight meals to slow cooked weekend feasts, beef's versatility lends itself to all occasions. This chapter will explore ways to prepare simple yet satisfying beef dishes to enjoy on a nose-to-tail carnivore lifestyle.

Seared Ribeye with Herb-Butter

Ribeye steaks contain the perfect marbling balance to deliver rich, beefy flavor along with a tender, melt-in-your-mouth texture. Searing over high heat followed by basting in herb butter makes ribeyes worthy of any special occasion.

Ingredients:

2 bone-in ribeye steaks, cut 1-1 1/2 inches thick (about 2 pounds total)

4 tablespoons butter, softened

2 cloves garlic, minced

2 tablespoons fresh parsley, chopped

1 teaspoon fresh thyme leaves, chopped

1/4 teaspoon sea salt

Freshly ground black pepper

Instructions:

Remove steaks from the fridge and allow them to come closer to room temperature, about 20-30 minutes. Pat dry. Season liberally with salt and pepper.

Melt 2 tbsp butter in a cast iron skillet over high heat until foamy. Swirl to coat the pan.

Add steaks and sear undisturbed for 2 minutes per side. Use tongs to lift and check for a deep brown crust.

Add garlic to the pan and baste steaks with melted butter for 1 minute per side.

Remove steaks to a plate and top each with another tablespoon of butter. Tent foil to rest for 5 minutes.

Meanwhile, combine parsley, thyme, salt and pepper in the skillet butter. Swirl and drizzle over rested steaks before serving.

Slow Cooked Grass-Fed Beef Pot Roast

Slow cooking well-marbled chuck roast transforms the inexpensive cut into fall-apart tender pot roast perfection. Simple preparation plus hands-off cooking makes this a fuss-free family meal.

Ingredients:

3-4 lb grass-fed chuck roast

2 tsp sea salt

1 tsp black pepper

1 tsp dried thyme

1 small yellow onion, sliced

4 cloves garlic, minced

1 cup beef bone broth

Instructions:

Season roast all over with salt, pepper and thyme. Let sit for 10 minutes to absorb the flavor.

Heat a large Dutch oven over medium high heat. Brown roast on all sides, about 8 minutes total. Remove the roast.

Add onion and garlic to the pot, scraping any browned bits. Sauté 1 minute.

Return roast to pot along with broth. Bring to a simmer.

Cover and transfer to a 250°F oven. Cook for 3-4 hours until fork tender.

Remove roast to plate or cutting board. Let rest for 10 minutes then slice across the grain.

Meanwhile, use an immersion blender to purée onion, garlic and juices in a pot for gravy.

Coffee and Coriander Seared Flank Steak Salad

Flank steak delivers a big beefy flavor, especially when kicked up with spices and coffee rub. Sliced over spinach with creamy avocado, it creates a satisfying yet light carnivore meal.

Ingredients:

1 lb grass-fed flank steak

2 tsp ground coriander

2 tsp ground coffee

1 tbsp olive oil

1 avocado, sliced

5 oz fresh spinach

2 tbsp red wine vinegar

1/4 cup olive oil

Salt and pepper to taste

Instructions:

Mix coriander, coffee and 1 tbsp oil. Coat steak all over. Let marinate for 20 minutes.

Heat a grill or cast iron skillet over high heat. Sear steak 2-3 minutes per side for medium rare.

Rest steak 5 minutes then slice against the grain into thin strips.

Make vinaigrette by whisking vinegar and 1/4 cup olive oil.

Toss spinach with vinaigrette and divide among plates.

Top spinach with steak strips and avocado slices. Season with salt and pepper to serve.

Simple Ground Beef Meatballs

Ground meat offers a budget-friendly way to enjoy beef's nutrition in easy, everyday meals. These Greek-seasoned meatballs require just a few ingredients. Serve over zucchini noodles or cauliflower rice for a satisfying carnivore dinner.

Ingredients:

1 lb ground grass-fed beef

1 egg

2 cloves garlic, minced

1/4 cup minced onion

2 tsp dried oregano

1 tsp dried parsley

1/2 tsp sea salt

1/4 tsp ground pepper

2 tbsp olive oil

Instructions:

Mix all ingredients except oil in a bowl until just combined. Form into 16 meatballs.

Heat oil in a skillet over medium high heat. Add meatballs in a single layer. Fry turning occasionally until browned all over, about 8 minutes.

Transfer meatballs to a baking sheet. Bake at 400F for 5 minutes until cooked through.

Serve with pan sauce of choice or on top of non-starchy vegetables.

Bone Marrow Butter Seared Burgers

Bone marrow gives these indulgent burger patties an extra dose of nutrition and rich flavor. Browning the butter enhances the beefiness while keeping them tender. Top with cheese or bacon for the ultimate carnivore treat.

Ingredients:

1 lb ground beef (85% lean)

2 tbsp butter

2 tbsp bone marrow, finely diced

1 tsp Worcestershire sauce

1 tsp garlic powder

½ tsp onion powder

¼ tsp sea salt

Pepper to taste

2 tbsp ghee for frying

Instructions:

Mix all ingredients gently in a bowl until just combined. Form into 4 patties, about ½ inch thick. Make a shallow dent in the center to prevent puffing.

Melt ghee in a cast iron skillet over medium-high heat. When hot, add patties and fry 2-3 minutes per side for medium doneness.

Top each patty with a slice of cheese during the last minute of frying, if desired.

Remove burgers to a plate and let rest 1-2 minutes before serving on bunless lettuce wraps or with cauliflower buns.

Beef Heart and Bacon Skewers

Heart and other organ meats provide an inexpensive way to incorporate nutrient-dense variety into your carnivore plan. Grilling tenderizes the heart while bacon adds smoky flavor to these crowd-pleasing skewers.

Ingredients:

1 beef heart, sliced into 1-inch cubes

8 slices sugar-free bacon, cut in half

Bamboo or metal skewers

1 tbsp olive oil

1 tsp paprika

½ tsp garlic powder

½ tsp onion powder

¼ tsp sea salt

Black pepper to taste

Instructions:

Soak bamboo skewers in water for 30 minutes if using.

Toss heart cubes with oil, spices and seasonings. Marinate 15 minutes.

Weave heart cubes and bacon strips alternately onto skewers.

Grill over medium-high heat, turning occasionally until bacon crisps and heart cooks through, about 8-10 minutes.

Remove skewers to a platter and serve warm with extra salt and pepper.

Chapter 4:

Pork Recipes

Pork offers a tasty and versatile alternative to beef in carnivore cooking. Nutritionally, pork from heritage breed pigs raised on pasture rivals grass-fed beef, providing high-quality protein with anti-inflammatory omega-3 fatty acids. This chapter features recipes to enjoy pork for everyday meals or celebratory roasts.

Bacon-Wrapped Pork Tenderloin

Tenderloin's leanness gets balanced by bacon's fat and smoky flavor in this impressive yet easy recipe. Perfect for holidays or date nights, the sweet and savory pork pairs deliciously with cauliflower mash on the side.

Ingredients:

1 whole pork tenderloin, about 1 lb

6 slices sugar-free bacon

2 tbsp avocado oil

1 tbsp honey

2 tsp apple cider vinegar

1 tsp mustard powder

1/2 tsp smoked paprika

1/2 tsp sea salt

Instructions:

Mix oil, honey, vinegar, mustard, paprika and salt for glaze. Reserve 2 tbsp for serving.

Coat tenderloin all over with remaining glaze. Wrap bacon slices evenly around the top 2/3 of meat.

Roast at 400F for 25-30 minutes until bacon is crisp and meat registers 145F internally.

Rest 5 minutes then slice. Drizzle with reserved glaze before serving.

Pulled Pork Shoulder with Dry Rub

Smoky dry rubbed pulled pork makes carnivore versions of tacos, sandwiches and bowls easy. Slow cooking tougher shoulder cuts renders out amazingly tender, fall-apart meat that soaks up seasonings.

Ingredients:

1 boneless pork butt/shoulder, about 3 lbs

1/4 cup smoked paprika

2 tbsp garlic powder

1 tbsp onion powder

1 tbsp mustard powder

1 tbsp sea salt

1 tsp black pepper

1/2 tsp cayenne pepper (optional)

Instructions:

Mix all spices together for dry rub. Coat pork shoulder evenly on all sides.

Place pork in a slow cooker and cook on Low setting for 8-10 hours until extremely tender.

Remove pork to a large dish. Shred using two forks pulling meat apart.

Toss with pan juices to moisten. Serve wrapped in lettuce leaves or over cauliflower rice.

Crispy Pork Belly Burnt Ends

Pork belly burnt ends deliver crispy, charred meat candy flavor bombs. A sweet and spicy rub caramelizes into an irresistible crust when roasted low-and-slow. Serve these savory morsels over a salad or cauliflower mash.

Ingredients:

1-2 lbs pork belly, cut into 2-inch cubes

¼ cup erythritol or monk fruit sweetener

2 tbsp smoked paprika

1 tsp garlic powder

1 tsp onion powder

1 tsp sea salt

½ tsp cayenne pepper

Instructions:

Mix dry ingredients to form rub. Coat pork belly pieces all over.

Bake at 250F for 2 hours until tender. Drain excess fat if needed.

Increase heat to 400F. Roast 30 minutes more until cubes char and caramelize.

Enjoy pork belly burnt ends as finger food or over non-starchy sides.

Maple Sage Breakfast Sausage Patties

DIY sausage is easy with ground pork and breakfast staple spices. Forming into patties makes a quick, mess-free way to cook them. Freeze extras to reheat for fast protein any time of day.

Ingredients:

1 lb ground pork

1 tsp sea salt

½ tsp sage

½ tsp ground fennel

¼ tsp garlic powder

¼ tsp onion powder

¼ tsp maple flavoring or erythritol

⅛ tsp crushed red pepper flakes

Instructions:

Mix all ingredients gently but thoroughly in a bowl. Form into 8 equal patties.

Fry in a skillet over medium-high heat until browned on both sides and cooked through, about 4-5 minutes per side.

Serve with fried eggs or bake into breakfast sandwiches using large collard green leaves as buns.

Crispy Pork Rinds Nachos

Crunchy, no-carb pork rinds replace tortilla chips for guilt-free nachos that satisfy cravings. Pile on pulled pork, avocado, jalapeños, and all your favorite nacho toppings to create a carnivore feast.

Ingredients:

4 cups pork rinds

1 cup pulled pork

1 avocado, sliced or mashed

½ cup salsa verde

2 tbsp minced onion

1 jalapeño, sliced (optional)

¼ cup chopped cilantro

Lime wedges for serving

Instructions:

Spread pork rinds on a baking sheet in a single layer.

Top with pulled pork, avocado, salsa, onion, jalapeño, and cilantro.

Bake at 400F for 6-8 minutes until heated through.

Squeeze fresh lime juice over pork rinds nachos before devouring.

Chapter 5:

Lamb Recipes

Lamb delivers a nice change of pace from beef and pork in carnivore cooking. The rich, gamey flavor pairs beautifully with Mediterranean herbs and spices. Lamb provides protein, zinc, iron and B-vitamins on par with other red meats. This chapter highlights tasty ways to prepare lamb cuts for family meals or date nights.

Rosemary Crusted Lamb Chops

Quick-cooking lamb rib or loin chops cook to juicy perfection when coated in an aromatic rosemary crust. Searing and then roasting gives a crisp external crust while keeping interior meat tender. Serve these impressive yet easy chops with grilled asparagus spears.

Ingredients:

8 bone-in lamb rib chops or 4 lamb T-bone chops

2 tbsp olive oil

2 tbsp fresh rosemary, minced

4 garlic cloves, minced

1 tsp lemon zest

1/2 tsp sea salt

1/4 tsp black pepper

Instructions:

Combine oil, rosemary, garlic, lemon zest, salt and pepper.

Coat lamb chops all over with herb mixture. Let stand for 10 minutes.

Heat grill or skillet over high heat. Sear chops 2-3 minutes per side.

Transfer to a baking sheet and roast at 400F for 5 more minutes until browned and tender.

Rest chops 3 minutes before serving with pan drippings spooned over the top.

Braised Lamb Shanks with Tomatoes

Slow braising transforms tough lamb shanks into fall-off-the-bone tender delights. Tomato sauce lends a touch of richness and Mediterranean flair. Serve these succulent shanks over zucchini noodles or cauliflower rice.

Ingredients:

4 lamb shanks

2 tbsp olive oil

1 onion, diced

5 garlic cloves, minced

28 oz crushed tomatoes

1 cup chicken broth

2 tbsp tomato paste

1 tsp dried oregano

1 tsp dried basil

1 bay leaf

1/2 tsp sea salt

Freshly ground black pepper

Instructions:

Heat oil in a Dutch oven over medium high heat. Brown lamb shanks on all sides, about 8 minutes total. Remove shanks and set aside.

Add onion to the pot and cook until soft, about 5 minutes. Add garlic and cook for 1 minute more.

Return shanks to the pot along with remaining ingredients. Bring to a boil.

Reduce heat. Simmer covered for 2-3 hours until meat is falling off the bone.

Discard bay leaves. Shred meat off bones and mix with braising liquid before serving.

Merguez Lamb Sausages

Spicy North African merguez sausages pack big flavor into an easy handheld meal. Ground lamb provides the base while smoky paprika and warming spices like cumin and cinnamon shine. Grill or pan fry these exotic sausages any night of the week.

Ingredients:

1 lb ground lamb

1 tbsp smoked paprika

2 tsp ground cumin

1 tsp ground coriander

½ tsp cinnamon

½ tsp cayenne pepper

¼ tsp ground allspice

2 garlic cloves, minced

1 tbsp fresh mint, chopped

1 tsp sea salt

½ tsp black pepper

Instructions:

In a bowl, mix all ingredients until thoroughly combined.

Divide mixture into 8 equal parts. Roll each into sausage shapes about 5-6 inches long.

Heat a grill or skillet to medium high. Cook sausages, turning occasionally until browned all over and cooked through, about 8-10 minutes.

Serve sausages on their own or in lettuce leaf wraps with tahini sauce and pickled red onions.

Ground Lamb Kofta Kebabs

Ground lamb gets seasoned with bold spices and formed onto skewers for flavorful, portable kebabs. Grilling or broiling gives these middle eastern koftas irresistible char while keeping them juicy inside. Pair with tzatziki or tahini sauce for dipping.

Ingredients:

1 lb ground lamb

1 small onion, finely minced

3 cloves garlic, minced

1 tsp ground cumin

1 tsp ground coriander

½ tsp cinnamon

¼ tsp allspice

¼ tsp cayenne pepper

¼ cup chopped parsley

Sea salt and black pepper to taste

Instructions:

In a bowl, gently mix all ingredients until thoroughly combined. Refrigerate for 30 minutes.

Divide mixture into 8 equal portions. Press each portion evenly onto metal or pre-soaked bamboo skewers.

Grill or broil kebabs, turning occasionally, 6-8 minutes until cooked through.

Serve lamb kofta kebabs on a bed of salad or with tahini lemon drizzle.

Minted Lamb Lettuce Wraps

These easy lettuce wraps provide a refreshing one-bowl meal with Mediterranean flair. Quick-cooking ground lamb gets seasoned with mint, lemon and garlic for a light yet satisfying lunch or dinner.

Ingredients:

1 lb ground lamb

¼ cup minced onion

3 garlic cloves, minced

1 tbsp fresh mint, chopped

1 tsp lemon juice

½ tsp lemon zest

½ tsp sea salt

¼ tsp black pepper

8-12 large lettuce leaves

½ cucumber, sliced

1 tomato, diced

¼ cup crumbled feta cheese

Instructions:

Cook lamb and onion in a skillet over medium heat until browned and cooked through, about 6-8 minutes. Drain excess fat.

Remove from heat and stir in garlic, mint, lemon juice, lemon zest, salt and pepper.

Serve lamb mixture wrapped inside lettuce leaves topped with cucumber, tomato and feta.

Chapter 6:

Poultry Recipes

Chicken, turkey, duck and other birds offer lean protein options for carnivore meal planning variety. Poultry provides complete nutrition including B-vitamins, selenium, zinc and bioavailable amino acids. This chapter features nutritious poultry dishes to add to your regular recipe rotation.

Whole Roasted Chicken with Herbs

Nothing satisfies like a juicy roasted chicken. Coating it in an herb butter mixture makes the skin ultra crispy while keeping meat moist and infusing delicious flavor throughout. Enjoy this classic whole or use leftovers all week long in other meals.

Ingredients:

1 whole chicken, 4-5 pounds

4 tbsp butter, softened

1 tbsp fresh thyme leaves

1 tbsp fresh rosemary, chopped

2 tsp lemon zest

2 garlic cloves, minced

1 tsp paprika

¾ tsp sea salt

¼ tsp black pepper

Instructions:

Pat chicken dry. Loosen skin from meat without totally detaching it.

Mix all other ingredients to form a paste. Rub herb mixture evenly under skin.

Truss chicken and tie legs together. Place breast side up on a roasting pan.

Roast at 400F for 1-1 ¼ hours until skin browns and meat registers 165F.

Let rest 10 minutes before carving. Serve with pan juices spooned over the top.

Chicken Thigh Lettuce Wraps

Chicken thighs offer juicy, flavorful dark meat at an affordable price. Quick-cooking ground thigh meat wrapped in crunchy lettuce makes a perfect high-protein lunch or light dinner the whole family will love.

Ingredients:

1 lb ground chicken thigh

¼ cup minced onion

2 garlic cloves, minced

1 tsp fresh ginger, minced

1 tbsp coconut aminos

1 tsp sesame oil

1 tbsp rice wine vinegar

1 tsp erythritol

8-12 butter lettuce leaves

¼ cup chopped cashews

Sesame seeds for garnish

Instructions:

Cook ground chicken with onion and garlic in a skillet over medium heat until browned, about 6 minutes. Drain excess fat.

Remove skillet from heat and mix in ginger, coconut aminos, sesame oil, rice wine vinegar and erythritol.

Serve chicken mixture wrapped inside lettuce leaves topped with cashews and sesame seeds.

Buffalo Chicken Jalapeño Poppers

These kicked-up poppers pack all the flavors of hot wings into an easy, crowd-pleasing appetizer. Filling spicy cream cheese into jalapeños then coating in hot sauce and crisp bacon makes a perfect game day snack.

Ingredients:

12 large jalapeño peppers, halved lengthwise, seeds removed

4 oz cream cheese, softened

2 oz shredded pepper jack cheese

¼ cup hot sauce

¼ tsp garlic powder

¼ tsp onion powder

12 slices sugar-free bacon, halved

½ lb cooked chicken, shredded

Instructions:

Mix cream cheese, shredded cheese, hot sauce and spices until thoroughly blended.

Fill jalapeño halves evenly with cream cheese mixture. Top with shredded chicken.

Wrap each stuffed pepper with a half slice of bacon. Secure with a toothpick if needed.

Bake at 400F for 18-20 minutes until bacon crisps and filling browns slightly.

Chicken Pecan Pesto Zoodles

Vibrant pesto and toasted nuts dress up simple zucchini noodles for a light, fresh tasting chicken dish. Using thigh or breast meat balances the zoodles' lower carb count with satisfying protein. This makes an easy weeknight dinner the whole family can enjoy.

Ingredients:

3 cups zucchini noodles

½ lb cooked chicken breast or thigh, shredded

¼ cup pesto

2 tbsp toasted pecans, chopped

1 tbsp olive oil

1 garlic clove, minced

¼ tsp red pepper flakes

Sea salt and black pepper to taste

Instructions:

Heat a skillet with oil over medium. Add zoodles and sauté 1-2 minutes until just tender but still al dente. Remove from heat.

Add shredded chicken, pesto, pecans, garlic and red pepper flakes. Toss to thoroughly coat zoodles.

Season with salt and black pepper. Serve chicken pesto zoodles warm or chilled.

Turkey Meatloaf with Bacon and Cheese

This clever loaf incorporates cheese and bacon directly inside for bursts of flavor in every bite. Ground turkey provides a lean yet satisfying base while herbs and spices keep it moist. Sliced meatloaf served over greens makes a stellar meal.

Ingredients:

1 lb ground turkey (93% lean)

3 slices sugar-free bacon, finely chopped

½ cup shredded cheddar cheese

½ onion, minced

1 egg

¼ cup almond flour

1 tbsp Italian seasoning

2 garlic cloves, minced

1 tsp sea salt

¼ tsp black pepper

Instructions:

Mix all ingredients by hand in a large bowl until thoroughly combined.

Transfer mixture to a loaf pan and shape into a compact rectangular loaf.

Bake uncovered at 375F for 45 minutes until cooked through and browned. Insert a knife to check doneness.

Let meatloaf rest 5 minutes before slicing to serve.

Crispy Duck Leg Confit

Confit transforms tough duck legs into fall-off-the-bone tender, succulent meat infused with its own rendered duck fat. Serve crispy duck with a fruit compote or green salad for an elegant yet easy special occasion meal.

Ingredients:

4 duck leg quarters

2 tbsp dried thyme

1 tsp dried rosemary

12 garlic cloves, peeled and smashed

½ cup rendered duck fat or olive oil

Sea salt and pepper

Instructions:

Rinse and thoroughly pat dry duck legs. Season with thyme, rosemary and salt and pepper.

Place duck legs in a baking dish. Scatter garlic cloves around them and pour over duck fat.

Cover and cook at 300F for 2-3 hours until extremely tender.

Uncover and increase temperature to 400F. Cook 30 minutes more to crisp the skin.

Serve crispy duck legs with pan drippings and garlic cloves spooned over the top.

Chapter 7:

Wild Game and Exotic Meats

Beyond everyday beef, pork and chicken, some carnivores like to incorporate venison, bison, elk, boar and other game meats for variety. These wild protein sources offer unique nutritional profiles and bolder, richer flavors. This chapter explores recipes to cook less common meat varieties.

Coffee-Crusted Venison Backstrap

Venison backstrap provides incredibly lean and tender meat. A quick pan sear retains moisture while an aromatic coffee rub enhances the flavor. Serve alongside roasted asparagus spears for a satisfying meal.

Ingredients:

2 venison backstrap steaks, about 1 lb total

1 tbsp butter

2 tsp ground coffee

1 tsp garlic powder

1 tsp onion powder

1/2 tsp sea salt

1/4 tsp black pepper

Instructions:

Mix ground coffee and spices together. Coat steaks all over with rub.

Melt butter in a cast iron skillet over medium-high heat. Add steaks and cook to desired doneness, about 3 minutes per side for medium-rare.

Rest venison for 5 minutes before slicing across the grain to serve.

Elk Tenderloin Tips with Mushroom Cream Sauce

Quick-cooking elk tenderloin gets a rich flavor boost from an easy mushroom cream sauce. Browning the meat builds a savory fond that thickens the silky sauce. Pairs wonderfully with roasted broccoli or cauliflower.

Ingredients:

1 lb elk tenderloin, cut into 1-inch pieces

2 tbsp butter, divided

8 oz sliced mushrooms

3 cloves garlic, minced

1/2 cup beef bone broth

1/4 cup heavy cream

2 tsp Dijon mustard

1 tsp thyme

Salt and pepper to taste

Instructions:

Pat elk pieces dry and season with salt and pepper.

Heat 1 tbsp butter in a skillet over medium-high heat. Brown elk pieces for 1-2 minutes on each side. Remove meat and set aside.

Add remaining butter, mushrooms and garlic to the skillet. Sauté 3-4 minutes until softened.

Stir in broth and scrape any browned bits. Simmer until reduced by half, about 2-3 minutes.

Stir in cream, mustard, thyme and season with salt and pepper. Return the elk pieces to the skillet and simmer for 2 minutes more.

Serve elk tenderloin tips coated in the rich mushroom cream sauce.

Coffee-Chili Bison Burgers

Lean yet flavorful ground bison provides the base for these unique, satisfying burgers. A combo of spicy chili powder with mellow coffee gives them a bold kick. Load them into lettuce wraps with all your favorite fixings.

Ingredients:

1 lb ground bison

¼ cup minced onion

1 tbsp coffee grounds

2 tsp chili powder

1 tsp garlic powder

1 tsp sea salt

½ tsp black pepper

Avocado, bacon, cheese for topping

Instructions:

In a large bowl, gently mix all ingredients until just combined. Form into 4 patties.

Grill burgers or pan fry in a cast iron skillet 3-4 minutes per side until cooked to desired doneness, about medium.

Rest patties briefly before loading into lettuce leaf buns with desired toppings.

Cider Braised Wild Boar Ribs

Tough but flavorful wild boar ribs become fall-off-the-bone tender when slowly braised in apple cider. The sweet and savory sauce lacquers each meaty rib for finger-licking goodness.

Ingredients:

3 lbs wild boar ribs

1 onion, sliced

1 cup apple cider

½ cup chicken broth

2 tbsp apple cider vinegar

1 tbsp Dijon mustard

1 tsp dried sage

½ tsp dried thyme

Sea salt and black pepper to taste

Instructions:

Pat ribs dry and season with salt and pepper. Sear in batches in a skillet over high heat until browned. Transfer to a slow cooker.

Add remaining ingredients to the slow cooker. Cook on low setting for 7-8 hours.

Remove ribs carefully to serve the dish. Strain and defat braising liquid.

Bring liquid to a simmer and reduce until thickened into glaze, about 10 minutes.

Brush ribs with glaze before serving. Goes great with cauliflower mash.

Venison Liver Pâté

Nutrient-dense liver gets transformed into a smooth, savory spread. Venison liver provides a mildly gamey flavor while bacon and herbs balance it out. Enjoy with slices of fresh radish or endive for an upscale appetizer.

Ingredients:

8 oz venison liver, membranes removed

4 slices bacon, chopped

1 shallot, roughly chopped

2 garlic cloves

2 tbsp brandy

1 tsp fresh thyme

½ tsp ground nutmeg

½ tsp sea salt

¼ tsp black pepper

Instructions:

In a skillet over medium heat, sauté bacon until crispy, about 5 minutes. Remove and set aside.

Raise heat to high and quickly sear liver pieces 1-2 minutes on each side.

In a food processor, blend liver, shallot, garlic and brandy until smooth. Add 2 tbsp bacon fat from the skillet.

Pulse in remaining bacon pieces, thyme, nutmeg, salt and pepper until combined but still chunky.

Transfer to ramekins and chill covered at least 2 hours before serving. Garnish with extra thyme.

Chapter 8:

Organ Meats and Variety Cuts Recipes

Beyond typical steaks and chops, using organ meats and underappreciated cuts expands your carnivore cuisine horizons. Nutrient-dense liver, mineral-rich bone marrow, succulent short ribs and more offer budget-friendly variety. This chapter features recipes to savor nose-to-tail meat diversity.

Beef Heart Skewers with Chimichurri

Grilling tenderizes heart meat while infusing it with smoky flavor. Herbed chimichurri sauce enhances the beefiness. Try these skewers and discover how tasty hearts can be!

Ingredients:

1 beef heart, trimmed and cut into 1-inch cubes

1 cup parsley, chopped

¼ cup olive oil

3 tbsp red wine vinegar

4 garlic cloves, minced

1 shallot, minced

1 tbsp oregano, chopped

½ tsp red pepper flakes

Lime wedges, for serving

Sea salt and black pepper, to taste

Instructions:

Whisk together parsley, olive oil, vinegar, garlic, shallot, oregano and red pepper flakes. Season with salt and pepper. Set chimichurri sauce aside.

Thread beef heart cubes onto soaked bamboo skewers. Brush with oil and season with salt and pepper.

Grill skewers over medium-high heat, turning occasionally until cooked through, 8-10 minutes.

Serve beef heart skewers warm with chimichurri sauce drizzled over the top and lime wedges.

Pan Seared Beef Marrow Bones Appetizer

Marrow bones offer a mineral-rich addition to your carnivore diet. Roasting enhances their beefy flavor. Spread the bone marrow on celery sticks or crackers for an elevated appetizer.

Ingredients:

8 small beef marrow bones, about 3 inches long

Sea salt and black pepper

Celery sticks

Parsley, chopped for garnish

Instructions:

Preheat the oven to 425°F. Place marrow bones upright on a foil-lined baking sheet.

Roast 20-25 minutes until bones are browned and marrow is softened.

Cool slightly. Use a small spoon to scoop marrow out of bones and onto celery sticks.

Season with sea salt, black pepper and chopped parsley before serving.

Grass-Fed Beef Liver Pâté

Smooth, savory liver pâté makes an elegant appetizer for dinner parties. Nutrient-dense beef liver provides the base while bacon and heavy cream balance its distinctive flavor.

Ingredients:

1 lb grass-fed beef liver, cleaned, trimmed and cut into 1-inch pieces

4 slices sugar-free bacon, chopped

1 small shallot, chopped

3 garlic cloves, chopped

3 tbsp butter

3 tbsp heavy cream

2 tsp fresh thyme, chopped

½ tsp nutmeg

Sea salt and black pepper, to taste

Instructions:

Cook bacon in a skillet until crispy. Remove and set aside. Raise heat to high. Add liver and cook briefly until browned but still pink inside, about 2 minutes per side.

Transfer liver to a food processor. Add shallot, garlic, butter, cream, thyme and nutmeg. Puree until very smooth, scraping down sides.

Add crispy bacon and pulse a few times to retain some texture. Season with salt and pepper.

Transfer to ramekins, chill for at least 2 hours. Serve garnished with thyme and crackers.

Sous Vide Tri-Tip with Cilantro Chimichurri

Tender, flavorful tri-tip gets dressed to impress with a bright, herby cilantro chimichurri. Precision sous vide cooking followed by a quick sear maximizes moisture.

Ingredients:

2 lb grass-fed tri-tip roast

1 cup cilantro leaves, chopped

¼ cup olive oil

3 tbsp red wine vinegar

1 jalapeño, seeded and minced

3 garlic cloves, minced

½ tsp oregano

½ tsp cumin

Sea salt and black pepper, to taste

Instructions:

Blend cilantro, olive oil, vinegar, jalapeño, garlic, oregano and cumin. Season with salt and pepper. Refrigerate until ready to use.

Season tri-tip all over with salt and pepper. Vacuum seal and cook sous vide at 130°F for 2-4 hours until tender.

Remove meat from bag and pat dry thoroughly. Sear in a hot skillet or on a grill, 1-2 minutes per side to brown the exterior.

Let rest for 5 minutes then slice thinly across the grain. Serve drizzled with cilantro chimichurri.

Slow Cooker Oxtail Stew with Bacon and Mushrooms

Economical oxtail becomes fall-apart tender after a long braise. Bacon and cremini mushrooms add extra richness to this comforting stew. Enjoy ladled over mashed turnips or rutabaga.

Ingredients:

3 lbs oxtail pieces

6 slices sugar-free bacon, chopped

1 onion, diced

4 cloves garlic, minced

12 oz cremini mushrooms, quartered

2 cups beef bone broth

1 tbsp tomato paste

2 tsp thyme

1 bay leaf

2 tbsp arrowroot starch

Sea salt and black pepper, to taste

Instructions:

Pat oxtail pieces dry and season with salt and pepper. Sear in a skillet over high heat until well browned on all sides.

Transfer to a slow cooker along with bacon, onion, garlic, mushrooms and broth. Stir in tomato paste, thyme and bay leaf.

Cook on low setting for 6-8 hours until the meat is very tender and falling off the bone.

Remove bay leaves. Mix arrowroot with 2 tbsp cold water. Stir into stew to thicken slightly before serving.

Chapter 9:

Condiments, Sides and Drinks

While meat takes center stage, fun condiments, savory sides and suitable beverages round out delicious carnivore meals. This chapter offers recipes to make flavor-boosting sauces, zero-carb "side dishes," and low-carb drink options to complement your meat-focused cuisine.

Compound Butters

Flavored compound butters lend a flavor punch to steaks, chicken, fish and more. Letting them chill allows flavors to meld beautifully. Try these combos:

Lemon Herb Butter - Soften 4 tbsp butter. Mix in 1 tbsp minced parsley, 1 tsp lemon zest, 1 crushed garlic clove, and a pinch of salt.

Blue Cheese Bacon Butter - Soften 4 tbsp butter then mix in 2 tbsp crumbled blue cheese, 2 slices cooked and chopped bacon, and 1/4 tsp black pepper.

Everything Bagel Butter - Soften 4 tbsp butter then mix in 1 tsp dried onion flakes, 1 tsp poppyseeds, 1 tsp sesame seeds, ½ tsp garlic powder, and ¼ tsp salt.

Chipotle Lime Butter - Soften 4 tbsp butter then mix in juice and zest of 1 lime, 1 tsp adobo sauce from canned chipotles, and pinch of cayenne pepper.

Rosemary Sea Salt Butter - Soften 4 tbsp butter then mix in 2 tsp minced fresh rosemary, 1 crushed garlic clove, and ¼ tsp quality sea salt.

Let flavored butters chill for at least 30 minutes to allow flavors to meld. Form into log shapes, wrap in parchment and refrigerate for up to 2 weeks. Slice off pats as needed to top meats or vegetables.

Simple Pan Creamy Jus

This easy sauce turns pan drippings into an elegant, creamy gravy with only a few ingredients. Simmering concentrates flavors while arrowroot starch gently thickens.

Ingredients:

2 tbsp pan dripping or fat

1 shallot, minced

1 garlic clove, minced

1 cup beef bone broth

¼ cup heavy cream

1 tbsp arrowroot starch

1 tsp thyme leaves

Salt and pepper to taste

Instructions:

After cooking the meat, pour off the drippings into a saucepan. Leave 2 tbsp fat in the pan.

Add shallot and garlic to the pan drippings. Sauté 1 minute over medium heat.

Whisk in broth, heavy cream and arrowroot starch. Simmer for 5 minutes until slightly thickened.

Stir in thyme and any browned bits scraped from the pan. Season with salt and pepper before serving sauce over steaks, roasts or chops.

Simple Horseradish Cream

Whipping horseradish into whipped cream tames its bite while still providing that signature zing. Serve this easy cream alongside beef or fish like salmon.

Ingredients:

½ cup heavy whipping cream

2 tbsp prepared horseradish

1 tsp Dijon mustard

½ tsp lemon juice

Pinch of sea salt

Instructions:

Using a hand mixer or stand mixer, whip heavy cream until it holds stiff peaks, about 2-3 minutes.

Fold in prepared horseradish, Dijon, lemon juice and salt until just combined.

Transfer to a serving bowl or ramekins. Refrigerate for up to 5 days.

Chunky Chimichurri Sauce

This fresh herb sauce adds big flavor to everything from grilled meats to eggs and even vegetables. Make a batch to keep on hand for quick meals anytime.

Ingredients:

2 cups parsley leaves, chopped

½ cup olive oil

1/4 cup red wine vinegar

4 garlic cloves, minced

1 shallot, minced

2 tbsp oregano, chopped

1 tsp red pepper flakes

½ tsp sea salt

¼ tsp black pepper

Instructions:

Combine all ingredients in a bowl and mix thoroughly. Taste and adjust acidity or seasoning as desired.

Store chimichurri sauce in the refrigerator for up to 1 week. Remove 30 minutes before using to take the chill off.

Use as a marinade, drizzle for grilled meats, or even toss with non-starchy veggies.

Mushroom Gravy

Earthy mushroom flavor gives this gravy a big umami taste without any starch or flour. Low carb and nutritious, it's terrific over chicken, pork chops, steak and more.

Ingredients:

½ oz dried mushrooms

½ cup boiling water

1 tbsp butter

8 oz cremini mushrooms, sliced

1 shallot, minced

2 garlic cloves, minced

1 ½ cups chicken broth

½ tsp thyme

Salt and pepper to taste

Instructions:

Combine dried mushrooms with ½ cup boiling water. Let stand for 10 minutes to rehydrate. Drain, reserving liquid.

Melt butter in a skillet over medium-high heat. Add cremini mushrooms and sauté 5 minutes.

Add shallot, garlic, rehydrated mushrooms and cook 2 minutes more.

Stir in reserved mushroom soaking liquid, chicken broth, and thyme. Simmer until reduced by half, about 8-10 minutes.

Puree mushroom gravy using an immersion blender or regular blender. Season to taste.

Creamy Horseradish Sauce

This easy blender sauce packs all the flavor of classic steakhouse horseradish cream but lighter. Greek yogurt provides a tangy base while keeping it dairy-free.

Ingredients:

½ cup plain Greek yogurt

3 tbsp prepared horseradish

1 tbsp lemon juice

1 tbsp olive oil

1 tsp Dijon mustard

1 garlic clove, minced

¼ tsp sea salt

¼ tsp black pepper

Instructions:

Add all ingredients to a blender. Blend until completely smooth and combined.

Taste and adjust salt, pepper or horseradish to suit your preference.

Transfer to a serving bowl or container. Refrigerate for up to 1 week.

Serve alongside grilled meats like steak, pork chops, brisket or prime rib.

Cauliflower Rice Three Ways

Riced cauliflower makes a low carb base to flavor just about any way you like. Here are three tasty options:

Basic: Pulse cauliflower florets in a food processor until rice-like consistency. Heat 1 tbsp oil in a skillet over medium heat. Sauté riced cauliflower 3-5 minutes until tender but still al dente. Season with salt and pepper.

Mexican Style: Follow basic instructions but add 1 tbsp taco seasoning along with cauliflower to the skillet.

Cheesy: Follow basic instructions but stir in 1/4 cup shredded cheddar or cream cheese once cauliflower is cooked. Cover and let melt 1 minute before serving.

For all variations, add cooked chicken, beef or other protein to turn "rice" into a meal.

Zucchini Noodle Puttanesca

Spiralized zucchini noodles provide a perfect low carb vehicle for this boldly-flavored olive puttanesca sauce. Topping with Parmesan cheese adds a savory finish.

Ingredients:

3 medium zucchinis, spiralized

1 tbsp olive oil

3 cloves garlic, minced

1 (14.5 oz) can diced tomatoes

1/4 cup kalamata olives, sliced

2 tbsp capers, drained and rinsed

1 tsp anchovy paste (optional)

1/4 tsp red pepper flakes

1/4 cup Parmesan cheese, grated

Instructions:

Heat olive oil in a large skillet over medium. Add garlic and sauté 1 minute.

Add diced tomatoes, olives, capers, anchovy paste and red pepper flakes. Simmer for 10 minutes.

Add spiralized zucchini noodles and gently toss to coat in sauce. Cook just until warmed through, about 2 minutes.

Remove from heat and top with grated Parmesan before serving.

Loaded Radishes

Make the most of radishes' natural peppery flavor by loading them up with tasty fat and toppings. Stuff with your favorite cheeses, herbs and meats for an easy carnivore side.

Ingredients:

1 bunch radishes, greens removed

2 oz cream cheese, softened

2 slices cooked bacon, chopped

1 tbsp fresh chives, chopped

½ tsp lemon juice

Sea salt and black pepper to taste

Instructions:

Rinse radishes and slice off the root end. Cut a thin slice off the top as well.

Mix together cream cheese, bacon bits, chives, lemon juice and salt and pepper.

Spoon cream cheese mixture into radish cavities.

Serve loaded radishes as finger food appetizers or alongside main dishes.

Keto Fat Bombs

Chapter 10:

Meal Plans and Prep Tips

Planning out recipes and preparing some components ahead of time helps make sticking to a carnivore diet easier. This chapter provides sample weekly meal plans along with batch cooking tips, storage tricks and advice for dining out and travel.

7-Day Carnivore Meal Plan

Planning meals ahead takes the guesswork out of carnivore eating. This sample week provides easy recipe ideas for breakfast, lunch and dinner:

Monday:

Breakfast: Bacon and egg cups

Lunch: Leftover pot roast wrapped in lettuce leaves

Dinner: Ribeye steak with roasted asparagus

Tuesday:

Breakfast: Ground sausage patties with fried eggs

Lunch: Sliced chicken breast salad with creamy horseradish dressing

Dinner: Pork tenderloin medallions with mushroom cream sauce

Wednesday:

Breakfast: Smoked salmon and scrambled eggs

Lunch: Tuna salad lettuce wraps with pickle spears

Dinner: Lamb kofta kebabs with cauliflower rice

Thursday:

Breakfast: Steak and egg breakfast bowl

Lunch: Chicken salad stuffed in celery sticks

Dinner: Venison backstrap with charred Brussels sprouts

Friday:

Breakfast: Bacon and goat cheese omelet

Lunch: Leftover lamb kebabs with radishes

Dinner: Crispy skin salmon with dill Hollandaise sauce

Saturday:

Breakfast: Cheese crisps with sliced deli meat

Lunch: Taco salad with ground beef

Dinner: Spatchcock chicken with broccoli slaw

Sunday:

Breakfast: Ham and fried egg cups

Lunch: Zucchini noodle chicken Alfredo

Dinner: Prime rib roast with horseradish cream

Batch Cooking Carnivore Proteins

Batch cooking proteins like chicken breasts, ground beef and sausage ahead of time makes assembling quick meals throughout the week effortless.

Roast or poach 4-6 chicken breasts at once. Shred meat for salads, wraps or reheated with sauces.

Brown 2+ pounds ground beef or lamb. Portion into meal sizes to add to veggie bowls or lettuce wraps.

Grill, bake or pan sear 1-2 pounds sausage patties or meatballs. Reheat as needed for breakfast or snacks.

Hard boil a dozen eggs. Keep refrigerated to enjoy on their own or incorporate into other dishes.

Roast tenderloin, whole chickens or pork loin. Shred or slice meat for multiple meals like soups, stir fries and omelets.

Keeping prepped proteins on hand removes any excuses for grabbing unhealthy convenience foods when hunger strikes.

Freezer Carnivore Meals

Preparing double batches of recipes to stock your freezer ensures you always have healthy options available:

Double meatloaf, meatballs or burgers. Wrap individually and freeze for up to 3 months. Defrost as needed in the refrigerator.

Make extra egg muffins or breakfast sausage patties. Keep frozen, warmed under broiler or toaster oven when ready to eat.

Cook two chickens at once. Shred and freeze portions in 1-2 cup bags for use in soups, wraps, casseroles etc.

Grill or pan sear extra steak or chops. Let cool completely, vacuum seal and freeze to pull out on busy nights.

A well-stocked carnivore freezer prevents falling off plan when you don't feel like cooking.

Tips for Convenient Cooking

Streamline meal prepping with these handy habits:

Dedicate 1 afternoon on weekends to prep recipes for the week ahead like breakfast egg bites and marinated proteins.

Use a slow cooker or Instant Pot for hands-off batch cooking. Toss in ingredients, set and forget.

Let the oven do the work. Roast multiple pounds of meat at once. Cook once, enjoy leftovers.

Prep is produced once when you get home from the grocery store. Wash, cut and store veggies to grab easily. Set up an always-stocked charcuterie board in the refrigerator. Keep sliced cheeses, cured meats, and mustard on hand for instant snacks.

Maintain a well-organized pantry with labeled containers so ingredients are easy to locate and use.

Prioritizing convenience encourages consistency when tackling any dietary pattern long-term.

Carnivore Diet Grocery Shopping Tips

Shopping smart helps you stick to carnivore eating while still stretching your budget:

Seek out sales and buy meat in bulk when discounted. Repackage into meal-size portions and freeze.

Join a warehouse store for discounts on bulk packages of meat, eggs and non-carb staples. Purchase with a friend if portions are too big.

Check for markdowns. Meat nearing sell-by dates is often 25-50% off. Cook soon or freeze immediately.

Buy whole cuts rather than pre-cut steaks or ground meat. You control portioning plus processed meats cost more.

Look for manager's specials on organ meats like liver and heart which are frequently discounted.

Purchase fattier cuts like ribeye, chuck roast, chicken thighs which offer more nutrition per pound.

With a little strategizing, eating carnivore style doesn't have to devastate your food budget.

Dining Out Carnivore

Don't isolate yourself socially just because you're eating carnivores. With a little planning, you can still meet friends for meals out:

Suggest steakhouses or Brazilian grill restaurants where you can get meat cooked simply. Ask for no sugary sauces.

Check the menu in advance online and scout carnivore-friendly options. Call ahead about modifications.

At burger places, ask for lettuce wrap in place of the bun and get toppings/condiments on the side.

Mexican restaurants load up on meat options like fajita chicken or steak without rice and beans. Ask for extra guacamole.

Many Italian restaurants will serve chicken parmesan or marsala without pasta if requested. Get a side salad instead.

If the menu has little you can eat, focus on protein like boneless wings or shrimp cocktail. Balance meals at home.

Be polite, not pushy, with special requests. With the right strategies, dining out doesn't have to derail your carnivore efforts.

Carnivore Diet Travel Tips

You needn't put your carnivore eating on pause when traveling. A little preparation makes staying on track easy:

Pack snacks like beef jerky, pork rinds, tuna pouches, cheese whisps and nuts when driving or flying.

Grill or oven-finish steaks or burgers when staying in vacation rentals. Pick up groceries locally to cook.

Research the nearest grocery store when you arrive at the hotel. Stock up on supplies like lunch meat, instant broth and snack bars.

For long flights, request lean protein menu items. Bring your own high-fat snacks like olives, nuts or avocado.

Scope out restaurant menus where you're visiting. Pick places with good steak, wings, burger and seafood options.

Explain diet to relatives or friends you're visiting and ask to keep meat, eggs and veggies on hand. Offer to bring dishes.

With smart preparation, sticking to a carnivore away from home doesn't have to be challenging at all.

Appendix:

Resources for Sourcing and Cooking Meat

To get the most out of an all-meat diet, seek out quality sources for procuring top-tier proteins along with helpful accessories for preparation and storage. Here are some useful resources to check out:

Local butcher shops offer customized cuts of high-quality meat from animals raised humanely on pasture. Building a relationship with a butcher can help you access specialty items.

Farmers markets provide opportunities to purchase grass-fed meats, pastured eggs and organ meats directly from regional producers. Try ordering whole or half animals for significant savings.

Online vendors like Butcher Box deliver free-range, sustainably sourced meats like heritage pork and grass-fed beef right to your door. Order once or subscribe.

Kitchen tools like meat slicers, grinders, thermometers, vacuum sealers and cast iron skillets greatly simplify preparing and preserving meat.

Stainless steel freezer containers allow you to safely store pre-portioned meat for months without risk of freezer burn.

Digital cooking resources include sous vide circulators along with Instant Pot and slow cookers for hands-off meat cooking with perfect results.

Equipping your kitchen properly and sourcing from ethical suppliers helps you follow the carnivore diet optimally for health.